YOUR KNOWLEDGE HAS VALUE

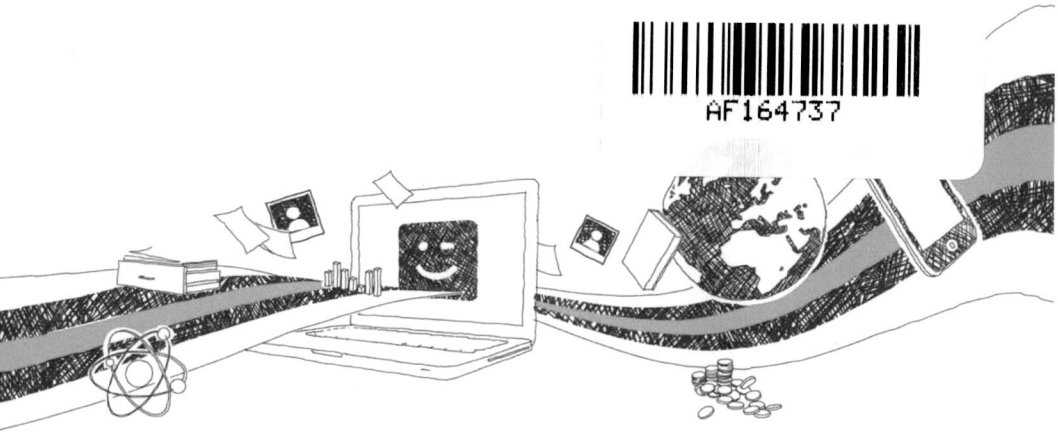

- We will publish your bachelor's and master's thesis, essays and papers

- Your own eBook and book - sold worldwide in all relevant shops

- Earn money with each sale

Upload your text at www.GRIN.com
and publish for free

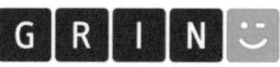

Bibliographic information published by the German National Library:

The German National Library lists this publication in the National Bibliography; detailed bibliographic data are available on the Internet at http://dnb.dnb.de .

This book is copyright material and must not be copied, reproduced, transferred, distributed, leased, licensed or publicly performed or used in any way except as specifically permitted in writing by the publishers, as allowed under the terms and conditions under which it was purchased or as strictly permitted by applicable copyright law. Any unauthorized distribution or use of this text may be a direct infringement of the author s and publisher s rights and those responsible may be liable in law accordingly.

Imprint:

Copyright © 2018 GRIN Verlag
Print and binding: Books on Demand GmbH, Norderstedt Germany
ISBN: 9783668648906

This book at GRIN:

https://www.grin.com/document/388761

Patrick Kimuyu

Implications of Virginia Henderson's Theory of Nursing

GRIN Verlag

GRIN - Your knowledge has value

Since its foundation in 1998, GRIN has specialized in publishing academic texts by students, college teachers and other academics as e-book and printed book. The website www.grin.com is an ideal platform for presenting term papers, final papers, scientific essays, dissertations and specialist books.

Visit us on the internet:

http://www.grin.com/

http://www.facebook.com/grincom

http://www.twitter.com/grin_com

OVERVIEW OF VIRGINIA HENDERSON'S BACKGROUND

- Virginia Avenel Henderson was born in Kansas City, in 1897.
- In 1921, she obtained her Diploma in Nursing from the Army School of Nursing in Washington D.C.
- She spent her first 2 years of practice at the Henry Street Visiting Nurse Service before moving to Norfolk Protestant Hospital in Virginia, in 1923, where she taught nursing (Petiprin, 2015).
- In 1929, she joined Columbia University where she obtained her Bachelor's Degree and Master's Degree in 1932 and 1934, respectively.
- After graduation, she taught at Columbia University until 1948. She then joined Yale University School of Nursing where she worked as a research associate.
- She died on 19 March, 1996 (Ahtisham & Jocaline, 2015).
- Henderson is regarded as the First Lady of Nursing because of her role in identifying the key concepts of disease prevention and health promotion (Burggraf, 2012).

HENDERSON'S BASIC METAPARADGMS

- Henderson developed the Need Theory out of influence by her nursing practice and education (Current Nursing, 2012).
- She then developed a satisfactory definition of nursing practice through the use of four major metaparadgms: Individual, Environment, Health, and Nursing.

- Individual
  - Basic needs form an integral component of health.
  - Mind and body are interrelated and inseparable.
  - A patient comprises of parts with biopsychosocial needs.
  - Considers sociological, psychological, spiritual, and biological components (Clares, Freitasm, Galiza & Almeida, 2012).
- Health
  - Health is defined on the basis of an individual's ability to meet physical, emotional and biological needs independently.
  - Nurses need to focus on disease prevention, cure and health promotion.

Environment

Figure removed due to copyright reasons

Figure 1: Illustration of environment (Geocaniga, Matias, Macha & Patayon, n.d.)

- Environment refers to external influences and conditions affecting life and development.
- Settings within which an individual lives.
- Community has impact on individual, as well as, the family.
- Nursing care enhance the patient's ability to perform the 14 components unaided.

Nursing

- Nursing care is meant to offer temporary assistance to a patient to satisfy the 14 basic needs.
- Nurse provides assistance and support to patients, in order to gain independence in performing life activities (Vandemark, 2006).
- Nurse serves as a scientific problem solver, hence requires knowledge.

THEORETICAL ASSERTIONS OF HENDERSON'S THEORY

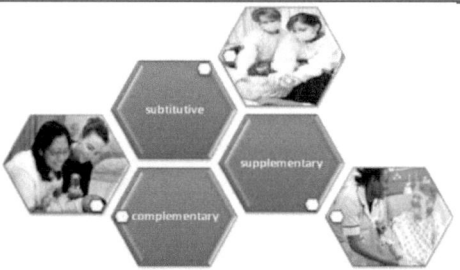

Figure 2: Nurse-Patient Relationship (Geocaniga et al., n.d.)

❖ Nurse-Patient Relationship
- Nursing care is meant to offer temporary assistance to a patient to satisfy the 14 basic needs.
- Nurse provides assistance and support to patients, in order to gain independence in performing life activities (Vandemark, 2006).
- Nurse serves as a scientific problem solver, hence requires knowledge.

- ❖ The Nurse-Physician Relationship
    - Henderson held the proposition that the function of nurses is independent from that of physicians.
    - She held that the plan of care is only implemented in a way that enhances therapeutic plan prescribed by the physician.
    - Nurses follow a philosophy that enables patients to receive orders from physicians.

- ❖ The Nurse as Healthcare Team Member
    - Henderson held that collaborative functioning by the healthcare team creates harmony in the provision of primary care.
    - As such, a nurse plays an integral role in the healthcare team.
    - As a member of the team, a nurse contributes by implementing the program of care.
    - Henderson emphasizes that each member in the team should carry out the respective roles and responsibilities interdependently.

IMPLICATIONS OF HENDERSON'S THEORY

- From a critical perspective, Henderson's theory bears immense implications for nursing practice, nursing education and nursing research.

Theory's Implications For Nursing Practice

- Implications of the theory for nursing practice are based on the 14 fundamental needs.
- The theory is highly significant in four main aspects of nursing practice: Assessment, Diagnosis, Planning, Implementation, and Evaluation as demonstrated by Ahtisham & Jocaline (2015) case study.

- ❖ Assessment: the assessment of the patient based on Henderson's 14 basic needs help in determining the lacking needs (Matt, 2014).
- ❖ Nursing diagnosis: Based on the 14 basic needs, it is possible to address the underlying factors contributing to the patient's illness.
- ❖ Nursing care plan: By using the 14 needs assessment results, nurses formulate the plan of care to complement the physicians prescribed plan.

- ❖ Implementation of nursing care plan:
  - It is apparent that Henderson's theory is reliable in the implementation of care plan.
  - It helps the sick to gain recovery from illness.
  - It also helps in providing assistance in maintaining health among well individuals (Ahtisham & Jocaline, 2015).

- ❖ Nursing evaluation:
  - The theory is useful for nursing evaluation.
  - For instance, it helps in determining whether nursing goals are achieved or not based on nursing definitions and laws that govern the nursing practice.

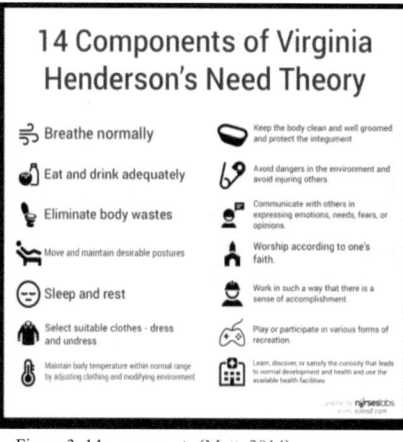

Figure 3: 14 components (Matt, 2014)

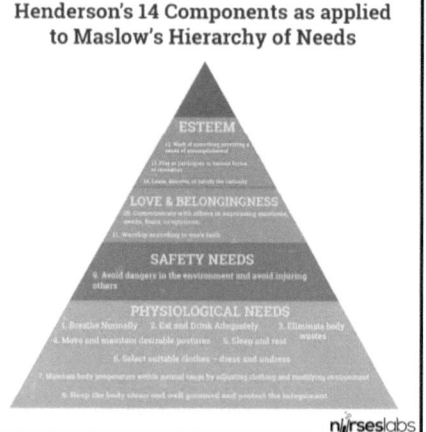

Figure 4: The relationship between Henderson's 14 components and Maslow's theory (Matt, 2014)

Theory's Implications For Nursing Education

- Similarly, Henderson's theory bears immense implications for nursing education.
- Foremost, the development of the nursing education curriculum is based on the theory's core concepts.
- The development of nursing education curriculum follows three main phases that ensure students' progress in the learning process.

- First, the curriculum provides students with fundamental skills for assisting patients to meet their basic needs and attain independence.
- Second, it can enable students to develop scientific inquiry skills by covering courses in social, biological and physical sciences.
- They also take courses in the field of humanities, in order to gain extensive knowledge of providing effective care in different settings.
- Third, the curriculum that has been developed using Henderson's theory engage students in studying the patient and all the 14 needs.

Theory's Implications For Nursing Research

- In the current perspective of nursing that focuses on evidence-based practice, Henderson's theory appears to be quite significant.

  - Foremost, the theory provides a comprehensive framework that is useful for developing new ideas and knowledge.

  - Second, the theory forms the basis for scientific inquiry.
  - For instance, the 14 components generate research questions that can be investigated to improve practice.

- In general, the theory's implications for nursing research are attributable to Henderson's emphasis on the significance of research in improving the nursing career.

THEORY'S STRENGTHS AND WEAKNESSES

- Henderson's theory can be critiqued from the perspective of its strengths and weaknesses.
- ❖ Strengths:
  - The widespread acceptance of Henderson's definition of nursing is attributable to it 14 components.
  - It is explicit that the 14 components make the theory simple and logical.
  - In addition, the theory does not have demographic restrictions such as age and gender.
  - It is applicable to individuals of all genders and ages (Matt, 2014).
- ❖ Weaknesses:
  - One of the greatest shortcomings of Henderson's theory is the lack of a conceptual framework. The 14 components of the theory are not interconnected through a conceptual diagram.
  - Second, the theory does not provide adequate explanation on the nurse's role in assisting the patient to achieve 'peaceful death.'

CONCLUSION

- Conclusively, it is apparent that Henderson achieved her goal in restructuring the definition of nursing through her theory.

- In retrospect, her principal focus on the basic human needs has led to a significant development of the nursing profession.

- It has widespread applications in the nursing practice, nursing education and nursing research.

- As such, the theory exhibits a holistic approach to all aspects of nursing.

- Moreover, Henderson's theory is widely accepted in the nursing practice due to the simplicity, logic and self-explanatory aspect of its 14 components of care.

REFERENCES

- Ahtisham, Y., & Jocaline, S. (2015). **Integrating nursing theory and process into practice; Virginia's Henderson need theory.** *International Journal of Caring Sciences,* 8(2), 443-450. Retrieved from http://www.internationaljournalofcaringsciences.org/docs/23_ahtisham.pdf
- Burggraf, V. (2012). **Overview and Summary: The New Millennium: Evolving and Emerging Nursing Roles.** *OJIN: The Online Journal of Issues in Nursing,* 17(2). DOI: 10.3912/OJIN.Vol17No02ManOS
- Clares, J., Freitasm, M., Galiza, F., & Almeida, P. (2012). **Sleep and rest needs of seniors: a study grounded in the work of Henderson.** *Acta paul. enferm.,* 25(1). Retrieved from http://www.scielo.br/scielo.php?script=sci_arttext&pid=S0103-21002012000500009
- Current Nursing (2012). **Virginia Henderson's need theory.** Retrieved from http://currentnursing.com/nursing_theory/Henderson.html
- Geocaniga, M., Matias, N., Macha, P., & Patayon, R. (n.d.). *Virginia Avenel Henderson: major concepts.* Retrieved from http://vhenderson2011.blogspot.co.ke/p/major-concepts.html
- Matt, V. (2014). **Virginia Henderson's nursing need theory.** Retrieved from http://nurseslabs.com/virginia-hendersons-need-theory/
- Petiprin, A. (2015). *Virginia Henderson - nursing theorist.* Retrieved from http://www.nursing-theory.org/nursing-theorists/Virginia-Henderson.php
- Vandemark, L.M. (2006). **Awareness of self & expanding consciousness: using Nursing theories to prepare nurse –therapists.** *Ment Health Nurs.,* 27(6), 605-15.

YOUR KNOWLEDGE HAS VALUE

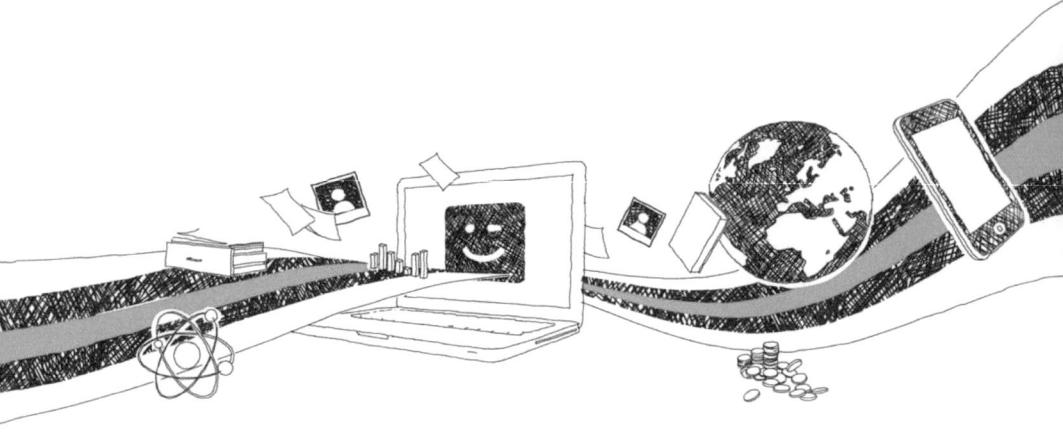

- We will publish your bachelor's and master's thesis, essays and papers

- Your own eBook and book - sold worldwide in all relevant shops

- Earn money with each sale

Upload your text at www.GRIN.com and publish for free

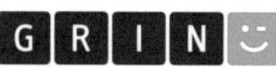